LOW FODMAP FOOD LIST

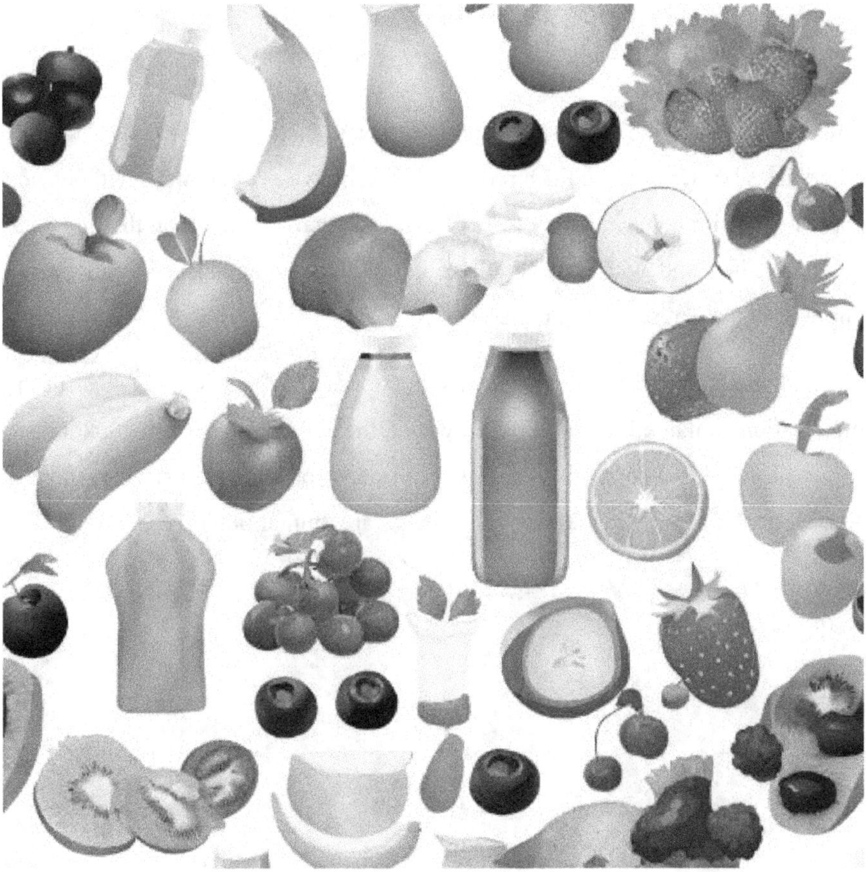

LYSANDRA QUINN

TABLE OF CONTENTS

INTRODUCTION

Have you ever experienced the frustration of a seemingly never-ending quest to find relief from digestive discomfort? I certainly have, and it was a moment of profound revelation that led me to embark on a journey that has culminated in the creation of this Low FODMAP Food List. As a dietician, my life's purpose has always been to help individuals find solace in the realm of nutrition, but the catalyst for this Endeavor was a deeply personal and transformative experience that I am excited to share with you.

It was a crisp autumn morning, the kind that fills your lungs with the promise of a new day. The golden leaves crunched under my feet as I made my way to my Favorite farmers' market. With each step, I couldn't help but feel a sense of anticipation in the air, almost as though the universe was conspiring to unveil a secret that had eluded me for years.

For as long as I could remember, I had been plagued by digestive issues. Bloating, cramps, and unpredictable bathroom visits were my constant companions. Over the years, I had seen countless doctors, tried various medications, and adhered to a multitude of dietary regimens, all in the hopes of finding the elusive answer to my discomfort. Yet, my condition remained an enigma, a persistent reminder that the path to wellness was obscured by a thick veil of confusion.

The farmers' market that day was teeming with vibrant produce, and I found myself drawn to a bustling stall adorned with a kaleidoscope of fruits and vegetables. The vendor, an elderly woman with a smile that radiated warmth, was passionately extolling the virtues of her organic wares to anyone who would listen. Intrigued, I approached her booth, and it was there that my life would change forever.

She handed me a beautifully illustrated pamphlet, which bore the enigmatic title: "Low FODMAP Diet - Unlocking Digestive Freedom." As I skimmed through its pages, the words seemed to leap off the paper, resonating with me in a way that nothing had before. The Low FODMAP diet was touted as a solution for individuals like me, those who had endured the torment of digestive issues for years on end.

FODMAPs, I discovered, were a group of fermentable carbohydrates found in many common foods. They had the potential to wreak havoc on the digestive system of those with sensitive bowels. The diet aimed to eliminate or reduce the intake of these troublesome substances, offering a lifeline to those who had been suffering in silence. I knew, in that moment, that I had stumbled upon something extraordinary.

I took the pamphlet home with me that day, and as I delved deeper into the world of Low FODMAP, I found myself increasingly captivated. The diet had been developed by researchers at Monash

University in Australia, and its effectiveness had been demonstrated in numerous clinical trials. The evidence was compelling, and I couldn't help but wonder why I had never come across this approach in my years of dietary study.

With newfound determination, I embarked on my own Low FODMAP journey. The transformation was nothing short of miraculous. My symptoms began to dissipate, and I found myself liberated from the constant discomfort that had held me captive for so long. It was as though a dark cloud had lifted, and the sun shone brighter than ever before.

My experience with the Low FODMAP diet was nothing short of a revelation, and it became clear to me that this knowledge had the potential to change countless lives. This was not just another fad diet; it was a scientifically validated approach to addressing the root causes of digestive distress. I knew I had to share this discovery with the world, and the idea for this book was born.

The Low FODMAP Food List is the culmination of years of research, personal experience, and a burning desire to help others find the relief and freedom that I had discovered. In these pages, you will find not only a comprehensive list of foods that are safe and suitable for those on a Low FODMAP diet, but also practical guidance on how to navigate the culinary landscape, create delicious meals, and regain control of your digestive health.

The journey to understanding the intricacies of the Low FODMAP diet has been both enlightening and humbling. It has reinforced my belief that the power of nutrition is boundless and that with the right information, we can transform our lives. I have seen the impact of this diet on my clients and witnessed their joy as they experience a newfound sense of well-being. This is the knowledge I want to impart to you, dear reader, so that you too can embark on your own journey towards digestive freedom.

As you turn the pages of this book, you'll discover the magic of the Low FODMAP diet, the stories of individuals whose lives have been forever changed by its principles, and the practical tools you need to embrace this transformative way of eating. It's my hope that, through these words, you will not only find a practical guide to navigating the world of Low FODMAP, but also a source of inspiration to take control of your own health.

So, whether you're a fellow sufferer of digestive distress, a healthcare professional seeking to expand your knowledge, or someone simply interested in the remarkable impact of nutrition on our lives, I invite you to join me on this journey. The Low FODMAP Food List is not just a book; it's a testament to the life-changing power of food and the boundless potential for healing that lies within our grasp.

Welcome to a world of digestive freedom. Let the adventure begin.

Chapter 1

Low FODMAP

FODMAPs, which stands for Fermentable Oligosaccharides, Disaccharides, Monosaccharides, and Polyols, are a group of carbohydrates found in various foods. These compounds are known to be poorly absorbed in the small intestine and can trigger digestive symptoms in some individuals. FODMAPs can be categorized into five main types:

Oligosaccharides: These include fructans and galacto-oligosaccharides (GOS) and are found in foods like wheat, rye, onions, garlic, and legumes.

Disaccharides: Lactose is the primary disaccharide, found in dairy products like milk, yogurt, and soft cheese.

Monosaccharides: Fructose, particularly in excess of glucose, can be problematic. It is present in various fruits like apples, pears, and honey.

Polyols: These are sugar alcohols such as sorbitol and mannitol, often found in some fruits and artificial sweeteners.

The Importance of a Low FODMAP Diet

A low FODMAP diet is essential for individuals with irritable bowel syndrome (IBS) and other gastrointestinal conditions. The primary goal of this diet is to reduce the intake of high-FODMAP foods to alleviate symptoms like bloating, abdominal pain, diarrhea, and constipation. By doing so, it helps manage these symptoms and improve overall digestive comfort. It is important to note that a low FODMAP diet is not a long-term solution but rather a diagnostic and short-term management strategy.

How to Use This Food List

When embarking on a low FODMAP diet, it's crucial to understand which foods are high and low in FODMAPs. This knowledge will help you make informed dietary choices. Here's a basic guide on how to use a FODMAP food list:

Identify High-FODMAP Foods: Consult a comprehensive FODMAP food list or work with a registered dietitian to identify foods high in FODMAPs. These are the foods that should be temporarily limited or eliminated from your diet.

Plan Your Meals: Once you've identified the high-FODMAP foods to avoid, plan your meals around low-FODMAP options. These can include rice, potatoes, carrots, and many meats, fish, and poultry.

Monitor Portion Sizes: Even some low-FODMAP foods may become problematic in large quantities. Pay attention to portion sizes to ensure you don't exceed your individual tolerance levels.

Gradual Reintroduction: After a period of strict low-FODMAP eating and symptom improvement, gradually reintroduce FODMAP-containing foods to identify your specific triggers. This is best done under the guidance of a healthcare professional.

Keep a Food Diary: Maintain a food diary to track your daily intake and any associated symptoms. This will help you and your healthcare provider make necessary adjustments.

Chapter 2

Low FODMAP Food Categorize

Low FODMAP Fruits

Blueberries

- Serving Size: 1 cup (148g)
- Calories: 84
- Carbohydrates: 21g
- Dietary Fiber: 3.6g
- Sugars: 9.7g

Strawberries

- Serving Size: 1 cup (144g)
- Calories: 46
- Carbohydrates: 11g
- Dietary Fiber: 3g
- Sugars: 7g

Raspberries

- Serving Size: 1 cup (123g)
- Calories: 64
- Carbohydrates: 15g
- Dietary Fiber: 8g
- Sugars: 5.4g

Cantaloupe

- Serving Size: 1 cup (160g)
- Calories: 54
- Carbohydrates: 14g
- Dietary Fiber: 1.6g
- Sugars: 13g

Kiwi

- Serving Size: 1 medium (100g)
- Calories: 61
- Carbohydrates: 15g
- Dietary Fiber: 2.1g
- Sugars: 9g

Pineapple

- Serving Size: 1 cup (165g)
- Calories: 83
- Carbohydrates: 22g
- Dietary Fiber: 2.3g
- Sugars: 16g

Oranges

- Serving Size: 1 medium (130g)
- Calories: 62
- Carbohydrates: 15g
- Dietary Fiber: 3g
- Sugars: 12g

Grapes

- Serving Size: 1 cup (151g)
- Calories: 104
- Carbohydrates: 27g
- Dietary Fiber: 1g
- Sugars: 23g

Honeydew Melon

- Serving Size: 1 cup (177g)
- Calories: 64
- Carbohydrates: 16g
- Dietary Fiber: 1.4g
- Sugars: 14g

Papaya

- Serving Size: 1 cup (140g)
- Calories: 55
- Carbohydrates: 14g
- Dietary Fiber: 2.5g
- Sugars: 9g

Grapefruit

- Serving Size: 1/2 medium (123g)
- Calories: 52
- Carbohydrates: 13g
- Dietary Fiber: 2g
- Sugars: 8g

Lemon

- Serving Size: 1 medium (58g)
- Calories: 17
- Carbohydrates: 5.4g
- Dietary Fiber: 1.6g
- Sugars: 1.5g

Lime

- Serving Size: 1 medium (67g)
- Calories: 20
- Carbohydrates: 7g
- Dietary Fiber: 2.1g
- Sugars: 1g

Clementines

- Serving Size: 1 medium (74g)
- Calories: 35
- Carbohydrates: 9g
- Dietary Fiber: 1.3g
- Sugars: 7g

Cranberries

- Serving Size: 1 cup (100g)
- Calories: 46
- Carbohydrates: 12g
- Dietary Fiber: 4.6g
- Sugars: 4g

Low FODMAP Vegetables

Carrots

- Serving Size: 1 medium (61g)
- Calories: 25
- Carbohydrates: 6g
- Dietary Fiber: 2g
- Sugars: 3g

Bell Peppers (Red)

- Serving Size: 1 cup (149g)
- Calories: 46
- Carbohydrates: 9g
- Dietary Fiber: 3g
- Sugars: 6g

Zucchini

- Serving Size: 1 medium (196g)
- Calories: 33
- Carbohydrates: 7g
- Dietary Fiber: 2g
- Sugars: 3g

Spinach

- Serving Size: 1 cup (30g)
- Calories: 7
- Carbohydrates: 1g
- Dietary Fiber: 1g
- Sugars: 0g

Kale

- Serving Size: 1 cup (67g)
- Calories: 33
- Carbohydrates: 6g
- Dietary Fiber: 1g
- Sugars: 0g

Cucumbers

- Serving Size: 1/2 cucumber (118g)
- Calories: 8
- Carbohydrates: 2g
- Dietary Fiber: 0.5g
- Sugars: 1g

Eggplant

- Serving Size: 1 cup (82g)
- Calories: 20
- Carbohydrates: 5g
- Dietary Fiber: 3g
- Sugars: 3g

Green Beans

- Serving Size: 1 cup (125g)
- Calories: 31
- Carbohydrates: 7g
- Dietary Fiber: 3g
- Sugars: 3g

Tomatoes (Cherry or Grape)

- Serving Size: 1 cup (149g)
- Calories: 27
- Carbohydrates: 6g
- Dietary Fiber: 2g
- Sugars: 4g

Bok Choy

- Serving Size: 1 cup (70g)
- Calories: 9
- Carbohydrates: 2g
- Dietary Fiber: 1g
- Sugars: 1g

Lettuce (Romaine)

- Serving Size: 1 cup (47g)
- Calories: 8
- Carbohydrates: 1g
- Dietary Fiber: 1g
- Sugars: 0g

Potatoes (Red)

- Serving Size: 1 medium (150g)
- Calories: 149
- Carbohydrates: 34g
- Dietary Fiber: 2g
- Sugars: 1g

Parsnips

- Serving Size: 1 cup (133g)
- Calories: 100
- Carbohydrates: 24g
- Dietary Fiber: 7g
- Sugars: 6g

Cabbage (Green)

- Serving Size: 1 cup (89g)
- Calories: 22
- Carbohydrates: 5g
- Dietary Fiber: 2g
- Sugars: 2g

Turnips

- Serving Size: 1 cup (130g)
- Calories: 36
- Carbohydrates: 8g
- Dietary Fiber: 2g
- Sugars: 4g

Low FODMAP Proteins

Chicken Breast

- Serving Size: 3 ounces (85g)
- Calories: 128
- Protein: 26g
- Total Fat: 2.7g
- Saturated Fat: 0.7g

Turkey

- Serving Size: 3 ounces (85g)
- Calories: 135
- Protein: 24g
- Total Fat: 3.1g
- Saturated Fat: 0.8g

Salmon

- Serving Size: 3 ounces (85g)
- Calories: 175
- Protein: 22g
- Total Fat: 9g
- Saturated Fat: 1.3g

Tuna

- Serving Size: 3 ounces (85g)
- Calories: 99
- Protein: 22g
- Total Fat: 0.5g
- Saturated Fat: 0.1g

Shrimp

- Serving Size: 3 ounces (85g)
- Calories: 84
- Protein: 18g
- Total Fat: 0.8g
- Saturated Fat: 0.2g

Tofu (Firm)

- Serving Size: 3 ounces (85g)
- Calories: 70
- Protein: 8g
- Total Fat: 4g
- Saturated Fat: 0.6g

Eggs

- Serving Size: 2 large eggs (100g)
- Calories: 143
- Protein: 12g
- Total Fat: 10g
- Saturated Fat: 3g

Pork (Tenderloin)

- Serving Size: 3 ounces (85g)
- Calories: 122
- Protein: 22g
- Total Fat: 3.4g
- Saturated Fat: 1.2g

Ground Beef (90% Lean)

- Serving Size: 3 ounces (85g)
- Calories: 184
- Protein: 21g
- Total Fat: 10g
- Saturated Fat: 4g

Cod

- Serving Size: 3 ounces (85g)
- Calories: 89
- Protein: 20g
- Total Fat: 0.7g
- Saturated Fat: 0.2g

Turkey Bacon

- Serving Size: 3 slices (57g)
- Calories: 135
- Protein: 11g
- Total Fat: 9g
- Saturated Fat: 2.6g

Lamb (Loin)

- Serving Size: 3 ounces (85g)
- Calories: 170
- Protein: 23g
- Total Fat: 7g
- Saturated Fat: 3.2g

Quail

- Serving Size: 1 quail (100g)
- Calories: 143
- Protein: 25g
- Total Fat: 5g
- Saturated Fat: 1.4g

Venison

- Serving Size: 3 ounces (85g)
- Calories: 135
- Protein: 23g
- Total Fat: 3g
- Saturated Fat: 1.1g

Lobster

- Serving Size: 3 ounces (85g)
- Calories: 76
- Protein: 16g
- Total Fat: 1g
- Saturated Fat: 0.2g

Low FODMAP Grains

Rice (White)

- Serving Size: 1 cup (195g)
- Calories: 205
- Carbohydrates: 45g
- Dietary Fiber: 0.6g
- Sugars: 0.1g

Quinoa

- Serving Size: 1 cup (185g)
- Calories: 222
- Carbohydrates: 39g
- Dietary Fiber: 5.2g
- Sugars: 1.6g

Oats (Gluten-Free)

- Serving Size: 1/2 cup (40g)
- Calories: 150
- Carbohydrates: 27g
- Dietary Fiber: 4g
- Sugars: 1g

Polenta (Cornmeal)

- Serving Size: 1 cup (160g)
- Calories: 152
- Carbohydrates: 32g
- Dietary Fiber: 2g
- Sugars: 0.3g

Buckwheat

- Serving Size: 1 cup (168g)
- Calories: 154
- Carbohydrates: 33g
- Dietary Fiber: 5g
- Sugars: 0.2g

Millet

- Serving Size: 1 cup (200g)
- Calories: 207
- Carbohydrates: 41g
- Dietary Fiber: 2.3g
- Sugars: 0.7g

Sorghum

- Serving Size: 1 cup (192g)
- Calories: 220
- Carbohydrates: 49g
- Dietary Fiber: 6.7g
- Sugars: 0.5g

Rice Noodles (Rice Vermicelli)

- Serving Size: 1 cup (174g)
- Calories: 192
- Carbohydrates: 44g
- Dietary Fiber: 0.8g
- Sugars: 0g

Cornflakes (Gluten-Free)

- Serving Size: 1 cup (28g)
- Calories: 100
- Carbohydrates: 24g
- Dietary Fiber: 0.9g
- Sugars: 3g

Buckwheat Noodles (Soba)

- Serving Size: 1 cup (114g)
- Calories: 113
- Carbohydrates: 23g
- Dietary Fiber: 2.7g
- Sugars: 0g

Rice Cakes (Plain)

- Serving Size: 1 rice cake (9g)
- Calories: 35
- Carbohydrates: 7g
- Dietary Fiber: 0g
- Sugars: 0g

Gluten-Free Bread

- Serving Size: 1 slice (28g)
- Calories: 80
- Carbohydrates: 16g
- Dietary Fiber: 0g
- Sugars: 1g

Corn Tortillas

- Serving Size: 1 tortilla (26g)
- Calories: 50
- Carbohydrates: 12g
- Dietary Fiber: 1g
- Sugars: 0g

Millet Flour

- Serving Size: 1 cup (119g)
- Calories: 409
- Carbohydrates: 87g
- Dietary Fiber: 7.6g
- Sugars: 2g

Rice Flour

- Serving Size: 1 cup (158g)
- Calories: 578
- Carbohydrates: 128g
- Dietary Fiber: 4.6g
- Sugars: 0.5g

Low FODMAP Dairy Alternatives

Lactose-Free Milk (e.g., lactose-free cow's milk)

- Serving Size: 1 cup (240ml)
- Calories: 90
- Carbohydrates: 12g
- Sugars: 12g
- Protein: 8g
- Fat: 0g

Almond Milk (Unsweetened)

- Serving Size: 1 cup (240ml)
- Calories: 13
- Carbohydrates: 1g
- Sugars: 0g
- Protein: 1g
- Fat: 1g

Rice Milk (Unsweetened)

- Serving Size: 1 cup (240ml)
- Calories: 113
- Carbohydrates: 27g
- Sugars: 0g
- Protein: 1g
- Fat: 1g

Coconut Milk (Canned, Unsweetened)

- Serving Size: 1 cup (240ml)
- Calories: 552
- Carbohydrates: 13g
- Sugars: 0g
- Protein: 5g
- Fat: 57g

Hemp Milk (Unsweetened)

- Serving Size: 1 cup (240ml)
- Calories: 60
- Carbohydrates: 1g
- Sugars: 0g
- Protein: 2g
- Fat: 5g

Lactose-Free Yogurt (e.g., lactose-free cow's milk yogurt)

- Serving Size: 1 cup (245g)
- Calories: 150
- Carbohydrates: 18g
- Sugars: 13g
- Protein: 11g
- Fat: 5g

Soy Milk (Unsweetened)

- Serving Size: 1 cup (240ml)
- Calories: 80
- Carbohydrates: 4g
- Sugars: 1g
- Protein: 7g
- Fat: 4g

Lactose-Free Cheese (e.g., lactose-free cheddar)

- Serving Size: 1 ounce (28g)
- Calories: 110
- Carbohydrates: 0g
- Sugars: 0g
- Protein: 7g
- Fat: 9g

Cashew Milk (Unsweetened)

- Serving Size: 1 cup (240ml)
- Calories: 25
- Carbohydrates: 1g
- Sugars: 0g
- Protein: 0g
- Fat: 2g

Macadamia Milk (Unsweetened)

- Serving Size: 1 cup (240ml)
- Calories: 50
- Carbohydrates: 1g
- Sugars: 0g
- Protein: 0g
- Fat: 5g

Lactose-Free Sour Cream

- Serving Size: 2 tablespoons (30g)
- Calories: 40
- Carbohydrates: 2g
- Sugars: 1g
- Protein: 0g
- Fat: 3.5g

Coconut Yogurt (Unsweetened)

- Serving Size: 1 cup (245g)
- Calories: 330
- Carbohydrates: 12g
- Sugars: 4g
- Protein: 2g
- Fat: 30g

Hazelnut Milk (Unsweetened)

- Serving Size: 1 cup (240ml)
- Calories: 35
- Carbohydrates: 1g
- Sugars: 0g
- Protein: 1g
- Fat: 3g

Pecan Milk (Unsweetened)

- Serving Size: 1 cup (240ml)
- Calories: 33
- Carbohydrates: 1g
- Sugars: 0g
- Protein: 0g
- Fat: 3g

Lactose-Free Ice Cream (e.g., lactose-free vanilla)

- Serving Size: 1/2 cup (66g)
- Calories: 120
- Carbohydrates: 16g
- Sugars: 8g
- Protein: 2g
- Fat: 6g

Low FODMAP Condiments and Spices

Salt

- Serving Size: 1 teaspoon (6g)
- Calories: 0
- Sodium: 2,300mg

Black Pepper

- Serving Size: 1 teaspoon (2g)
- Calories: 6
- Sodium: 0mg

Oregano (Dried)

- Serving Size: 1 teaspoon (1g)
- Calories: 3
- Sodium: 0mg

Thyme (Dried)

- Serving Size: 1 teaspoon (1g)
- Calories: 3
- Sodium: 0mg

Cumin (Ground)

- Serving Size: 1 teaspoon (2g)
- Calories: 7
- Sodium: 6mg

Chili Powder

- Serving Size: 1 teaspoon (2g)
- Calories: 8
- Sodium: 43mg

Basil (Dried)

- Serving Size: 1 teaspoon (1g)
- Calories: 3
- Sodium: 0mg

Paprika

- Serving Size: 1 teaspoon (2g)
- Calories: 8
- Sodium: 1mg

Turmeric (Ground)

- Serving Size: 1 teaspoon (2g)
- Calories: 8
- Sodium: 1mg

Cayenne Pepper

- Serving Size: 1 teaspoon (1g)
- Calories: 5
- Sodium: 1mg

Coriander (Ground)

- Serving Size: 1 teaspoon (2g)
- Calories: 6
- Sodium: 3mg

Parsley (Dried)

- Serving Size: 1 teaspoon (1g)
- Calories: 5
- Sodium: 6mg

Dill (Dried)

- Serving Size: 1 teaspoon (1g)
- Calories: 5
- Sodium: 5mg

Rosemary (Dried)

- Serving Size: 1 teaspoon (1g)
- Calories: 3
- Sodium: 2mg

Chives (Dried)

- Serving Size: 1 teaspoon (1g)
- Calories: 3
- Sodium: 0mg

Low FODMAP Snacks

Rice Cakes with Peanut Butter

- Serving Size: 2 rice cakes with 2 tablespoons of peanut butter
- Calories: 260
- Carbohydrates: 24g
- Protein: 7g
- Fat: 16g
- Sugars: 2g

Hard-Boiled Eggs

- Serving Size: 2 large eggs
- Calories: 140
- Protein: 12g
- Fat: 10g
- Carbohydrates: 1g
- Sugars: 1g

Cheddar Cheese Cubes

- Serving Size: 1 ounce (28g)
- Calories: 110
- Protein: 7g
- Fat: 9g
- Carbohydrates: 0g
- Sugars: 0g

Carrot Sticks with Hummus

- Serving Size: 1 cup of carrot sticks with 2 tablespoons of hummus.
- Calories: 100
- Carbohydrates: 15g
- Protein: 3g
- Fat: 4g
- Sugars: 3g

Rice Crackers with Tuna Salad

- Serving Size: 10 rice crackers with tuna salad
- Calories: 240
- Carbohydrates: 40g
- Protein: 14g
- Fat: 2g
- Sugars: 0g

Strawberries with Lactose-Free Yogurt

- Serving Size: 1 cup of strawberries with 1/2 cup of lactose-free yogurt
- Calories: 130
- Carbohydrates: 24g
- Protein: 6g
- Fat: 2g
- Sugars: 12g

Banana (Unripe)

- Serving Size: 1 medium unripe banana
- Calories: 105
- Carbohydrates: 27g
- Protein: 1g
- Fat: 0.3g
- Sugars: 14g

Almonds

- Serving Size: 1 ounce (28g)
- Calories: 160
- Carbohydrates: 6g
- Protein: 6g
- Fat: 14g
- Sugars: 1g

Popcorn (Plain, Air-Popped)

- Serving Size: 3 cups (24g)
- Calories: 93
- Carbohydrates: 19g
- Protein: 3g
- Fat: 1g
- Sugars: 0g

Cucumber Slices with Tzatziki

- Serving Size: 1 cup of cucumber slices with 2 tablespoons of tzatziki
- Calories: 60
- Carbohydrates: 9g
- Protein: 2g
- Fat: 2g
- Sugars: 3g

Grapes

- Serving Size: 1 cup (151g)
- Calories: 104
- Carbohydrates: 27g
- Protein: 1g
- Fat: 0g
- Sugars: 23g

Corn Chips (Plain)

- Serving Size: 1 ounce (28g)
- Calories: 140
- Carbohydrates: 15g
- Protein: 2g
- Fat: 8g
- Sugars: 0g

Pineapple Chunks

- Serving Size: 1 cup (165g)
- Calories: 83
- Carbohydrates: 22g
- Protein: 1g
- Fat: 0g
- Sugars: 16g

Baked Potato Chips

- Serving Size: 1 ounce (28g)
- Calories: 152
- Carbohydrates: 15g
- Protein: 2g
- Fat: 9g
- Sugars: 1g

Cantaloupe Slices

- Serving Size: 1 cup (160g)
- Calories: 54
- Carbohydrates: 14g
- Protein: 1g
- Fat: 0.3g
- Sugars: 13g

Low FODMAP Beverages

Water

- Serving Size: 1 cup (240ml)
- Calories: 0
- Carbohydrates: 0g
- Sugars: 0g

Peppermint Tea (Herbal)

- Serving Size: 1 cup (240ml)
- Calories: 0
- Carbohydrates: 0g
- Sugars: 0g

Green Tea

- Serving Size: 1 cup (240ml)
- Calories: 2
- Carbohydrates: 0g
- Sugars: 0g

Ginger Tea (Herbal)

- Serving Size: 1 cup (240ml)
- Calories: 5
- Carbohydrates: 1g
- Sugars: 0g

Chamomile Tea (Herbal)

- Serving Size: 1 cup (240ml)
- Calories: 2
- Carbohydrates: 0g
- Sugars: 0g

Lemonade (Made with Fresh Lemon Juice)

- Serving Size: 1 cup (240ml)
- Calories: 27
- Carbohydrates: 8g
- Sugars: 5g

Coconut Water

- Serving Size: 1 cup (240ml)
- Calories: 46
- Carbohydrates: 9g
- Sugars: 6g

Iced Coffee (Black)

- Serving Size: 1 cup (240ml)
- Calories: 2
- Carbohydrates: 0g
- Sugars: 0g

Orange Juice (Freshly Squeezed)

- Serving Size: 1 cup (240ml)
- Calories: 112
- Carbohydrates: 26g
- Sugars: 21g

Limeade (Made with Fresh Lime Juice)

- Serving Size: 1 cup (240ml)
- Calories: 112
- Carbohydrates: 28g
- Sugars: 25g

Rooibos Tea

- Serving Size: 1 cup (240ml)
- Calories: 0
- Carbohydrates: 0g
- Sugars: 0g

Almond Milk (Unsweetened)

- Serving Size: 1 cup (240ml)
- Calories: 13
- Carbohydrates: 1g
- Sugars: 0g

Cranberry Juice (100% Pure)

- Serving Size: 1 cup (240ml)
- Calories: 116
- Carbohydrates: 31g
- Sugars: 30g

Carrot Juice

- Serving Size: 1 cup (240ml)
- Calories: 80
- Carbohydrates: 18g
- Sugars: 13g

Grapefruit Juice (100% Pure)

- Serving Size: 1 cup (240ml)
- Calories: 96
- Carbohydrates: 23g
- Sugars: 22g

Chapter 3

High FODMAP to Avoid

Onions

- Serving Size: 1 medium onion (110g)
- Calories: 44
- Carbohydrates: 10g
- Sugars: 4g
- Fiber: 2g

Garlic

- Serving Size: 3 cloves (9g)
- Calories: 13
- Carbohydrates: 3g
- Sugars: 0g
- Fiber: 0g

Wheat-Based Bread

- Serving Size: 1 slice (28g)
- Calories: 68
- Carbohydrates: 13g
- Sugars: 1g
- Fiber: 1g

Apples

- Serving Size: 1 medium apple (182g)
- Calories: 95
- Carbohydrates: 25g
- Sugars: 19g
- Fiber: 4g

Pears

- Serving Size: 1 medium pear (178g)
- Calories: 51
- Carbohydrates: 13g
- Sugars: 9g
- Fiber: 5g

Watermelon

- Serving Size: 1 cup of diced watermelon (152g)
- Calories: 46
- Carbohydrates: 12g
- Sugars: 9g
- Fiber: 1g

Mushrooms

- Serving Size: 1 cup sliced (70g)
- Calories: 15
- Carbohydrates: 2g
- Sugars: 1g
- Fiber: 1g

Honey

- Serving Size: 1 tablespoon (21g)
- Calories: 64
- Carbohydrates: 17g
- Sugars: 17g
- Fiber: 0g

Cherries

- Serving Size: 1 cup (138g)
- Calories: 87
- Carbohydrates: 22g
- Sugars: 18g
- Fiber: 3g

Cauliflower

- Serving Size: 1 cup (100g)
- Calories: 25
- Carbohydrates: 5g
- Sugars: 2g
- Fiber: 2g

Black Beans

- Serving Size: 1 cup cooked (172g)
- Calories: 227
- Carbohydrates: 41g
- Sugars: 2g
- Fiber: 15g

Cashews

- Serving Size: 1 ounce (28g)
- Calories: 157
- Carbohydrates: 9g
- Sugars: 2g
- Fiber: 1g

Mango

Serving Size: 1 cup diced (165g)

- Calories: 150
- Carbohydrates: 38g
- Sugars: 32g
- Fiber: 3g

Lentils

- Serving Size: 1 cup cooked (198g)
- Calories: 230
- Carbohydrates: 40g
- Sugars: 3g
- Fiber: 16g

Milk (Regular)

- Serving Size: 1 cup (244g)
- Calories: 122
- Carbohydrates: 12g
- Sugars: 12g
- Protein: 8g

Cabbage

- Serving Size: 1 cup shredded (89g)
- Calories: 22
- Carbohydrates: 5g
- Sugars: 2g
- Fiber: 2g

Pistachios

- Serving Size: 1 ounce (28g)
- Calories: 156
- Carbohydrates: 8g
- Sugars: 2g
- Fiber: 3g

Cows Milk Cheese (e.g., cheddar)

- Serving Size: 1 ounce (28g)
- Calories: 110
- Carbohydrates: 1g
- Sugars: 0g
- Protein: 7g

Avocado

- Serving Size: 1/2 avocado (100g)
- Calories: 160
- Carbohydrates: 9g
- Sugars: 0.5g
- Fiber: 7g

Brussels Sprouts

- Serving Size: 1 cup (88g)
- Calories: 38
- Carbohydrates: 8g
- Sugars: 2g
- Fiber: 3g

CONCLUSION

As we draw the curtains on this journey through the world of Low FODMAP, I find myself filled with a deep sense of gratitude and hope. The stories shared, the knowledge imparted, and the path to digestive freedom we've explored together have been nothing short of inspiring. I hope that the pages you've just journeyed through have not only been a source of information but also a wellspring of hope and empowerment for you.

In the beginning, we embarked on this quest together with a shared understanding of the trials and tribulations that come with digestive discomfort. I, too, was once on that path, searching for answers and feeling the weight of my symptoms. But the discovery of the Low FODMAP diet was a turning point, a moment of revelation that set me on a course to help others. My own transformation fueled my passion to share this life-changing approach with you.

Throughout the pages of this book, we've delved deep into the science behind the Low FODMAP diet, explored the diverse range of foods that can be enjoyed, and learned how to navigate a world that may have once seemed overwhelming. We've celebrated the small victories, embraced the flavors of Low FODMAP cuisine, and marveled at the resilience of individuals who have discovered digestive freedom through this remarkable approach.

But our journey doesn't end here. It's only the beginning. As you close this book, I encourage you to carry the torch of knowledge and newfound awareness with you. The power to transform your digestive health lies in your hands, and the choices you make can lead to a life free from the chains of discomfort. It's a journey worth embarking upon, one that offers the promise of well-being, vitality, and the joy of savoring each moment without the shadow of digestive distress.

Remember, you are not alone on this path. There is a community of individuals who have walked the same road, and countless healthcare professionals who are ready to support you in your quest for better health. Seek their guidance, share your experiences, and become a part of a network that understands and encourages the pursuit of a life unburdened by the limitations of digestive issues.

I want to leave you with one powerful thought: Your health is your greatest wealth. The ability to live a life unencumbered by the debilitating effects of digestive discomfort is a precious gift. With the knowledge you've gained from this book, you have the tools to take control of your health and experience the world in a whole new light. This journey is a testament to the resilience of the human spirit and the transformative power of knowledge.

So, as you close this chapter and embark on your own path to digestive freedom, remember that the journey may have its twists and turns, but the destination is well worth the effort. Embrace the Low FODMAP way of life, savor the flavors of delicious, nourishing foods, and relish the newfound freedom that awaits you.

Thank you for allowing me to be a part of your journey, and may your life be filled with health, happiness, and the joys of a life well-lived. Here's to embracing the journey of digestive freedom and to a future filled with endless possibilities.

With heartfelt wishes for your well-being and success on your path.

BONUS

10 Low FODMAP Recipes

Grilled Chicken and Vegetable Skewers

Cooking Time: 20 minutes

Servings: 4

Ingredients:

- 1 pound (450g) chicken breast, cut into cubes.
- 1 zucchini, sliced into rounds.
- 1 red bell pepper, cut into chunks.
- 1 yellow bell pepper, cut into chunks.
- 1 tablespoon garlic-infused olive oil
- 1 tablespoon lemon juice
- Salt and pepper to taste

Instructions:

1. Preheat the grill to medium-high heat.
2. In a bowl, mix the garlic-infused olive oil, lemon juice, salt, and pepper.
3. Thread the chicken and vegetables onto skewers, alternating the pieces.
4. Brush the skewers with the oil and lemon mixture.

5. Grill for about 10 minutes, turning occasionally, until the chicken is cooked through and the vegetables are tender.

6. Serve hot.

Nutritional Information (per serving):

Calories: 180

Carbohydrates: 5g

Protein: 25g

Fat: 6g

Fiber: 2g

Quinoa and Roasted Vegetable Salad

Cooking Time: 30 minutes

Servings: 4

Ingredients:

- 1 cup quinoa
- 2 cups water
- 1 zucchini, sliced into rounds.
- 1 eggplant, cut into cubes.
- 1 red bell pepper, cut into chunks.
- 2 tablespoons garlic-infused olive oil
- 2 tablespoons balsamic vinegar
- Salt and pepper to taste

Instructions:

1. Preheat the oven to 400°F (200°C).
2. Toss the zucchini, eggplant, and red bell pepper with garlic-infused olive oil, balsamic vinegar, salt, and pepper.
3. Roast the vegetables for about 20 minutes, or until tender, stirring occasionally.
4. In a separate pot, cook the quinoa in water according to package instructions.
5. Once the quinoa and vegetables are cooked, mix them together in a large bowl.

6. Serve warm or at room temperature.

Nutritional Information (per serving):

- Calories: 260
- Carbohydrates: 48g
- Protein: 7g
- Fat: 6g
- Fiber: 9g

Baked Salmon with Lemon and Dill

Cooking Time: 20 minutes

Servings: 4

Ingredients:

- 4 salmon fillets
- 1 lemon thinly sliced.
- 2 tablespoons fresh dill, chopped.
- Salt and pepper to taste
- 2 tablespoons garlic-infused olive oil

Instructions:

1. Preheat the oven to 375°F (190°C).
2. Season the salmon fillets with salt, pepper, and dill.
3. Place lemon slices on top of each fillet.
4. Drizzle the garlic-infused olive oil over the salmon.
5. Bake for about 15-20 minutes, or until the salmon flakes easily with a fork.
6. Serve with your favorite low FODMAP side dish.

Nutritional Information (per serving):

Calories: 260

Carbohydrates: 1g

Protein: 27g

Fat: 17g

Fiber: 0g

Low FODMAP Spinach and Bacon Frittata

Cooking Time: 25 minutes

Servings: 4

Ingredients:

- 6 large eggs
- 1 cup spinach, chopped.
- 4 strips of cooked bacon, crumbled.
- 1/4 cup lactose-free milk
- Salt and pepper to taste
- 1 tablespoon garlic-infused olive oil

Instructions:

1. Preheat your oven to 350°F (175°C).
2. In a bowl, whisk together the eggs and lactose-free milk. Add salt and pepper.
3. Heat the garlic-infused olive oil in an oven-safe skillet over medium heat.
4. Add the spinach and sauté until wilted.
5. Pour the egg mixture into the skillet and sprinkle crumbled bacon on top.
6. Cook on the stovetop for a few minutes, then transfer the skillet to the oven.
7. Bake for about 15 minutes or until the frittata is set.

8. Slice and serve.

Nutritional Information (per serving):

Calories: 220

Carbohydrates: 1g

Protein: 15g

Fat: 17g

Fiber: 0g

Shrimp and Zucchini Noodles

Cooking Time: 20 minutes

Servings: 2

Ingredients:

- 8 oz (225g) shrimp peeled and deveined.
- 2 zucchinis, spiralized into noodles
- 1 tablespoon garlic-infused olive oil
- 1 tablespoon fresh basil, chopped.
- Salt and pepper to taste
- Red pepper flakes (optional)

Instructions:

1. Heat the garlic-infused olive oil in a pan over medium heat.
2. Add the shrimp and cook until they turn pink and opaque.
3. Remove the shrimp from the pan and set aside.
4. In the same pan, add the zucchini noodles and cook for a few minutes until slightly softened.
5. Season with salt, pepper, and red pepper flakes if desired.
6. Add the cooked shrimp and fresh basil to the zucchini noodles, toss to combine.
7. Serve hot.

Nutritional Information (per serving):

Calories: 190

Carbohydrates: 8g

Protein: 21g

Fat: 8g

Fiber: 2g

Baked Potato with Chives and Lactose-Free Sour Cream

Cooking Time: 45 minutes

Servings: 4

Ingredients:

- 4 medium-sized potatoes
- 2 tablespoons garlic-infused olive oil
- 2 tablespoons fresh chives, chopped
- Lactose-free sour cream (to taste)
- Salt and pepper to taste

Instructions:

1. Preheat your oven to 400°F (200°C).
2. Wash and scrub the potatoes, then pat them dry.
3. Pierce each potato with a fork a few times.
4. Rub the potatoes with garlic-infused olive oil, salt, and pepper.
5. Place the potatoes directly on the oven rack and bake for about 40-45 minutes or until tender.
6. Split the potatoes open and top with fresh chives and a dollop of lactose-free sour cream.

Nutritional Information (per serving):

Calories: 200

Carbohydrates: 40g

Protein: 4g

Fat: 3g

Fiber: 4g

Low FODMAP Sushi Rolls

Cooking Time: 30 minutes

Servings: 2

Ingredients:

- 2 nori seaweed sheets
- 1 cup sushi rice, cooked and seasoned with rice vinegar.
- 4 slices of cooked and peeled shrimp
- 1/2 cucumber thinly sliced.
- 2 tablespoons pickled ginger
- Soy sauce (gluten-free)
- Wasabi (optional)

Instructions:

1. Place a bamboo sushi rolling mat on a clean surface and cover it with plastic wrap.
2. Lay a nori sheet on the mat, shiny side down.
3. Wet your hands to prevent the rice from sticking and spread a thin layer of sushi rice over the nori, leaving about 1 inch uncovered at the top.
4. Add cucumber slices, cooked shrimp, and pickled ginger to the center of the rice.
5. Carefully roll up the nori sheet using the bamboo mat, applying gentle pressure.

6. Wet the top edge of the nori to seal the roll.

7. Slice the roll into bite-sized pieces.

8. Serve with gluten-free soy sauce and optional wasabi.

Nutritional Information (per serving):

Calories: 320

Carbohydrates: 68g

Protein: 10g

Fat: 1g

Fiber: 2g

Grilled Steak with Mashed Potatoes and Green Beans

Cooking Time: 35 minutes

Servings: 2

Ingredients:

- 2 steaks (your choice of cut)
- 4 medium-sized potatoes, peeled and cubed
- 1 cup green beans, trimmed
- 2 tablespoons garlic-infused olive oil
- Salt and pepper to taste
- Fresh rosemary (optional)

Instructions:

1. Preheat your grill to medium-high heat.
2. Rub the steaks with garlic-infused olive oil, salt, and pepper. If desired, add fresh rosemary for flavor.
3. Grill the steaks to your preferred doneness, about 4-5 minutes per side for medium-rare.
4. While the steaks are cooking, boil the potatoes until they are tender, then mash them with a little garlic-infused olive oil.
5. Steam the green beans until they are crisp-tender.

6. Serve the grilled steak with mashed potatoes and green beans.

Nutritional Information (per serving):

Calories: 450

Carbohydrates: 30g

Protein: 30g

Fat: 22g

Fiber: 5g

Low FODMAP Tuna Salad Wrap

Cooking Time: 15 minutes

Servings: 2

Ingredients:

- 1 can of canned tuna in water, drained
- 4 large lettuce leaves (as wraps)
- 1/2 cup shredded carrots
- 1/2 cup cucumber thinly sliced.
- 2 tablespoons mayonnaise (check for FODMAP-friendly ingredients)
- Salt and pepper to taste

Instructions:

1. In a bowl, combine the drained tuna, shredded carrots, and mayonnaise.
2. Season with salt and pepper.
3. Lay out the lettuce leaves and divide the tuna mixture among them.
4. Add cucumber slices on top of the tuna.
5. Fold the lettuce leaves to create wraps.
6. Serve immediately.

Nutritional Information (per serving):

Calories: 180

Carbohydrates: 6g

Protein: 20g

Fat: 9g

Fiber: 3g

Low FODMAP Omelet with Spinach and Tomatoes

Cooking Time: 15 minutes

Servings: 2

Ingredients:

- 4 large eggs
- 1 cup fresh spinach
- 1 small tomato, diced (remove seeds)
- 2 tablespoons garlic-infused olive oil
- Salt and pepper to taste

Instructions:

1. In a bowl, whisk the eggs and season with salt and pepper.
2. Heat garlic-infused olive oil in a non-stick skillet over medium heat.
3. Add the spinach and cook until wilted.
4. Add the diced tomatoes to the skillet and cook for another minute.
5. Pour the whisked eggs over the spinach and tomatoes in the skillet.
6. Cook until the omelet is set and the edges are golden brown.
7. Fold the omelet in half and serve.

Nutritional Information (per serving):

Calories: 220

Carbohydrates: 4g

Protein: 14g

Fat: 16g

Fiber: 2g

www.ingramcontent.com/pod-product-compliance
Lightning Source LLC
Chambersburg PA
CBHW050834260726
48660CB00006B/2238